I0702957

Menopause Weight Loss for Women

By Daphne Sinclair

Copyright © 2024 by Daphne Sinclair.

All rights reserved. No part of this publication may be reproduced, distributed, or transmitted in any form or by any means, including photocopying, recording, or other electronic or mechanical methods, without the prior written permission of the publisher, except for short quotes used in reviews and critical articles.

Medical Alert

The information contained in this book is intended for educational purposes only and is not a substitute for professional medical advice, diagnosis, or treatment. Always consult your physician or other qualified health care professional for advice about your health condition. Do not ignore or delay seeking professional medical advice because of content in this book.

Limitation of Liability Clause

The authors and the publisher are not responsible for any damage resulting from the use of the information contained in this book. All content is provided "as is," and we do not guarantee its completeness, accuracy, timeliness, or suitability for any particular purpose.

Disclaimers regarding Medical Substitutes

This book is not a substitute for medical consultation and is not intended to diagnose or treat medical conditions.

Translation and Adaptation Rights

All rights to translate, adapt, and modify the content of the book without the prior consent of the publisher are expressly prohibited.

Local Law Compliance Information

Readers living outside the country of publication should consult local regulations to ensure that the book's content complies with local legal and medical requirements.

Digital Distribution and Sharing Rights

This book may not be copied, electronically shared, or archived without the express written permission of the publisher.

Copyrights to Graphics and Other Content

Content in the book that is subject to the copyright of other people (e.g., graphics, photos) is used under license or with right permission and cannot be reproduced without obtaining the appropriate rights.

ISBN: 9798327101319

ISBN: 9798327117037

Contents

Chapter 1: Introduction

Menopause is a natural stage in every woman's life that brings many physical, emotional, and hormonal changes. For many women, this period is associated with challenges related to maintaining a healthy weight. The book "Menopause Weight Loss Book" aims to provide comprehensive information and practical advice on managing weight during menopause. In this chapter, we will explain the importance of a healthy weight during this period, understand what menopause is, what its symptoms are, and how it affects a woman's body.

The Importance of a Healthy Weight During Menopause

A healthy weight is crucial for overall health and well-being at any stage of life, but it has special significance during menopause. Here are a few reasons why maintaining a healthy weight during this time is so important:

- **Reducing the Risk of Chronic Diseases:** Overweight and obesity are risk factors for many chronic diseases, such as heart disease, type 2 diabetes, hypertension, stroke, and some types of cancer. Maintaining a healthy weight can reduce the risk of these conditions.

- **Alleviating Menopausal Symptoms:** Studies show that overweight women may experience more intense menopausal symptoms, such as hot flashes, night sweats, and sleep problems. Maintaining a healthy weight can help alleviate these symptoms.

- **Improving Mental Health:** A healthy weight can also impact mental well-being. Women who maintain a healthy weight often feel more confident and are less prone to depression and anxiety.

- **Supporting Bone Health:** During menopause, women are more susceptible to bone loss and osteoporosis. Maintaining a healthy weight through a proper diet and regular physical activity can support bone health.

Understanding Menopause: What It Is and What Are Its Symptoms

Menopause is a natural biological process that marks the end of a woman's menstrual cycles. It typically occurs between the ages of 45 and 55, though it can happen earlier or later. Menopause is diagnosed after 12 months of no menstrual periods.

Stages of Menopause

- **Perimenopause:** This transitional period before menopause can last from a few months to several years. It is characterized by irregular menstrual cycles and a gradual decline in hormone levels, mainly estrogen and progesterone. During this time, the first symptoms of menopause may appear.

- **Menopause:** This is the point at which a woman has not had a menstrual period for 12 consecutive months. It marks the end of fertility and a significant reduction in the production of sex hormones by the ovaries.

- **Postmenopause:** This is the period after menopause, during which symptoms may persist, but the body gradually adjusts to the new hormonal state. After a few years, symptoms usually subside.

Menopausal Symptoms

Menopausal symptoms can vary from woman to woman, but the

most common ones include:

- **Hot Flashes:** A sudden feeling of heat, often with reddening of the skin and sweating, lasting from a few seconds to several minutes. Hot flashes are one of the most characteristic symptoms of menopause.

- **Night Sweats:** Intense sweating during sleep, which can lead to sleep disturbances and daytime fatigue.

- **Sleep Problems:** Insomnia, frequent waking at night, and difficulty falling asleep are common during menopause.

- **Mood Changes:** Women may experience mood swings, irritability, anxiety, and depression. Hormonal changes affect neurotransmitters in the brain, which can lead to these symptoms.

- **Memory and Concentration Issues:** Some women notice problems with memory and concentration, which may be related to hormonal changes.

- **Vaginal Dryness and Sexual Problems:** A decrease in estrogen levels can lead to vaginal dryness, painful intercourse, and reduced libido.

- **Decreased Bone Density:** Menopause is associated with an increased risk of osteoporosis, as a decrease in estrogen affects bone mass.

- **Skin and Hair Changes:** Skin may become thinner and less elastic, and hair may thin out.

How Menopause Affects a Woman's Body

Menopause involves many changes in the body that impact a woman's health and well-being. Understanding these changes can help effectively manage symptoms and maintain health.

- **Hormonal System:** Menopause signifies a significant decrease in the production of sex hormones by the ovaries. Estrogen, progesterone, and testosterone affect many processes in the body, including metabolism, bone health, brain function, and cardiovascular health.

- **Metabolic System:** A decline in estrogen levels affects metabolism, which can lead to weight gain. Loss of muscle mass and a slowing metabolic rate are typical during menopause.

- **Cardiovascular System:** Estrogens have a protective effect on the heart and blood vessels. Their decrease increases the risk of cardiovascular diseases, such as coronary artery disease, hypertension, and stroke.

- **Skeletal System:** A decrease in estrogen levels leads to a reduction in bone density, increasing the risk of osteoporosis and fractures.

- **Nervous System:** Hormonal changes can affect neurotransmitters in the brain, leading to mood swings, depression, anxiety, and memory problems.

- **Skin and Hair:** A decrease in estrogen affects collagen production, leading to reduced skin elasticity and thinning hair.

- **Urogenital System:** Vaginal dryness, urinary tract infections, and urinary incontinence are common problems associated with menopause.

Menopause is a natural stage in every woman's life, associated with many hormonal, physical, and emotional changes. Maintaining a healthy weight during menopause is crucial for reducing the risk of chronic diseases, alleviating menopausal symptoms, improving mental health, and supporting bone health. Understanding menopause, its symptoms, and its impact on the body allows better management of this period and making informed decisions about a healthy lifestyle.

Chapter 2: Causes of Weight Gain During Menopause

Weight gain during menopause is a common issue faced by many women. Understanding the causes of this phenomenon is crucial for effective weight and health management during this period. Below is a comprehensive discussion of the various causes of weight gain during menopause.

1. Hormonal Changes

Estrogen

One of the main hormones associated with menopause is estrogen. During menopause, estrogen levels significantly drop, which has several key effects:

- **Reduced Metabolism:** Estrogen plays a significant role in regulating metabolism. A decrease in estrogen levels leads to a slower metabolic rate, meaning the body burns fewer calories.

- **Abdominal Fat Accumulation:** Low estrogen levels promote fat storage in the abdominal area. Abdominal fat is more closely linked to metabolic diseases such as type 2 diabetes and heart disease.

- **Insulin Resistance:** A decline in estrogen levels can lead to insulin resistance, making it difficult to regulate blood sugar levels and promoting weight gain.

Progesterone

Like estrogen, progesterone levels also drop during menopause. Progesterone has a diuretic effect, so its deficiency can lead to water retention, which may be mistaken for weight gain.

Testosterone

Although testosterone is primarily associated with men, it also plays an important role in a woman's body. During menopause, testosterone levels decrease, leading to reduced muscle mass and a slower metabolic rate, which contribute to weight gain.

2. Metabolic Changes

Slower Metabolism

Metabolism naturally slows with age, but menopause can accelerate this process. A slower metabolism means the body needs fewer calories to maintain basic life functions, making it easier to gain weight if calorie intake remains the same as before.

Loss of Muscle Mass

As we age, we naturally lose muscle mass, which is further exacerbated by the decrease in testosterone and estrogen levels. Muscles burn more calories than fat tissue, so reduced muscle mass lowers the metabolic rate and increases the risk of weight gain.

3. Changes in Physical Activity

Reduced Physical Activity

Many women reduce their physical activity during menopause for various reasons, such as joint pain, fatigue, or lack of time. Less physical activity means fewer calories burned, contributing to weight gain.

Sedentary Lifestyle

The modern lifestyle often involves long hours of sitting, both at work and at home. A sedentary lifestyle reduces calorie burning and can lead to weight gain.

4. Changes in Diet

Increased Appetite

Hormonal changes can increase appetite, especially for sweet and fatty foods. Higher levels of cortisol, the stress hormone, can also increase cravings and lead to unhealthy eating habits.

Higher Calorie Intake

Some women may consume more calories during menopause, often without realizing it. Changes in diet, such as more frequent takeout meals or larger portions, can lead to weight gain.

Increased Alcohol Consumption

Some women increase their alcohol intake during menopause, which is high in calories and can lead to weight gain. Alcohol also affects metabolism and can disrupt hormonal balance.

5. Emotional and Psychological Changes

Stress

Stress is common during menopause due to hormonal changes, sleep problems, hot flashes, and other symptoms. High stress levels increase cortisol, which promotes fat storage in the abdominal area and increases appetite.

Sleep Problems

Sleep problems, such as insomnia, are common during menopause. Lack of sleep affects hormones that regulate appetite (leptin and ghrelin), leading to increased cravings and weight gain.

Depression and Mood Swings

Hormonal changes can affect mood, leading to depression, anxiety, and mood swings. These emotional changes can influence eating habits, such as emotional eating, which contributes to weight gain.

6. Genetic Factors

Genetic Predisposition

Genetics play an important role in shaping our body type and ability to lose weight. Women with a family history of weight gain during menopause may find it challenging to maintain a healthy weight.

Obesity-Related Genes

Some genes can influence how the body stores fat and regulates appetite. Women with genetic predispositions to obesity may have difficulty maintaining a healthy weight during menopause.

7. Medical Factors

Medications

Certain medications, such as antidepressants, anticonvulsants, steroids, and antihypertensive drugs, can cause weight gain as a side effect.

Thyroid Disorders

Hypothyroidism is a condition where the thyroid does not produce enough hormones, leading to a slower metabolism and weight gain. Thyroid disorders are more common in women during menopause.

Metabolic Syndrome

Metabolic syndrome is a group of symptoms that increase the risk of heart disease, diabetes, and other health problems. These symptoms include abdominal obesity, high blood pressure, high blood sugar, and abnormal cholesterol levels.

Weight gain during menopause is the result of many factors, including hormonal, metabolic, dietary, emotional, genetic, and medical changes. Understanding these causes is crucial for effective weight and health management during this period. Adopting a healthy lifestyle, regular physical activity, a balanced diet, and stress management techniques can help alleviate menopause symptoms and maintain a healthy weight.

Chapter 3: Healthy Diet

A healthy diet is the foundation of well-being and effective weight management during menopause. Properly balanced meals provide essential nutrients, support hormonal health, and help alleviate menopausal symptoms. In this chapter, we will discuss the principles of healthy eating, introduce superfoods for menopause, and present five sample meal plans for the week.

Principles of Healthy Eating

1. **Variety:** Consume a wide variety of foods to provide your body with all the essential nutrients, including proteins, fats, carbohydrates, vitamins, and minerals.

2. **Caloric Balance:** Maintain a caloric balance tailored to your energy needs. Avoid both excessive calorie intake and deficits.

3. **Macronutrients:**

- **Protein:** Supports muscle building and regeneration. Good sources include lean meats, fish, eggs, dairy, legumes, and nuts.

- **Fats:** Healthy fats, such as those found in olive oil, avocado, nuts, and fatty fish, are important for proper hormonal function.

- **Carbohydrates:** Provide energy. Choose complex carbohydrates like whole grains, vegetables, and fruits.

4. Micronutrients:

- **Vitamins and Minerals:** Ensure adequate intake of vitamins and minerals such as calcium, vitamin D, magnesium, potassium, and B vitamins, which are especially important during menopause.
- **Fiber:** Consume plenty of fiber, which aids digestion and helps maintain a feeling of fullness. It can be found in fruits, vegetables, whole grains, and legumes.
5. **Hydration:** Drink an adequate amount of water to stay hydrated and support metabolic processes.
6. **Regular Meals:** Eat regular meals to maintain a steady energy level and avoid hunger pangs.
7. **Avoid Processed Foods:** Limit the intake of processed foods, simple sugars, and trans fats, which can exacerbate menopausal symptoms and lead to weight gain.

Superfoods for Menopause

Superfoods are nutrient-rich foods that have beneficial effects on health. Here are some superfoods that can support health during menopause:

Soy and Soy Products:

- **Benefits:** Contain phytoestrogens, which may help alleviate menopausal symptoms such as hot flashes and night sweats.
- **Examples:** Tofu, tempeh, edamame, soy milk.

Flaxseed:

- **Benefits:** Rich in lignans, which have estrogen-like effects. Also contains omega-3 fatty acids that support heart health.
- **Examples:** Add to yogurt, oatmeal, smoothies.

Fatty Fish:

- **Benefits:** Contain omega-3 fatty acids that support heart and brain health and may reduce inflammation.
- **Examples:** Salmon, mackerel, sardines.

Cruciferous Vegetables:

- **Benefits:** Contain compounds that support detoxification and may help with hormonal balance.
- **Examples:** Broccoli, cabbage, cauliflower, Brussels sprouts.

Nuts and Seeds:

- **Benefits:** Provide healthy fats, protein, and fiber. Can help maintain a feeling of fullness and support heart health.
- **Examples:** Almonds, walnuts, chia seeds, sunflower seeds.

Berries:

- **Benefits:** Rich in antioxidants that help combat free radicals and support heart health.
- **Examples:** Blueberries, raspberries, strawberries, goji berries.

Avocado:

- **Benefits:** Contains healthy fats that support heart and skin health. Rich in fiber and potassium.
- **Examples:** Add to salads, sandwiches, smoothies.
- **Examples:** Use as a base for salad dressings, for frying, and baking.

Sample Meal Plans for the Week

Here are five variations of sample meal plans for the week, which can be adjusted to individual needs and preferences.

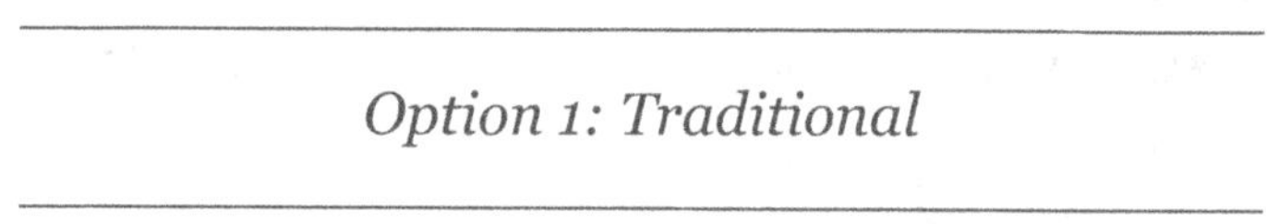

Option 1: Traditional

Monday

- Breakfast: Oatmeal with fruits, nuts, and flaxseed.
- Snack: Natural yogurt with honey and berries.
- Lunch: Chicken salad with avocado, tomatoes, and olive oil.

- Snack: Carrots and hummus.
- Dinner: Grilled salmon with broccoli and quinoa.

Tuesday

- Breakfast: Scrambled eggs with vegetables and whole grain bread.
- Snack: Nuts and dried fruits.
- Lunch: Lentil soup with vegetables.
- Snack: Celery sticks with peanut butter.
- Dinner: Baked turkey with quinoa and vegetables.

Wednesday

- Breakfast: Smoothie with kale, banana, berries, and almond milk.
- Snack: Chia seeds with yogurt and honey.
- Lunch: Whole grain pasta with tomato sauce, tofu, and spinach.
- Snack: Apple with almond butter.
- Dinner: Tuna salad with egg, olives, and vegetables.

Thursday

- Breakfast: Toast with avocado and poached egg.
- Snack: Smoothie with plant protein, spinach, and berries.
- Lunch: Stir-fry with shrimp, vegetables, and brown rice.

- Snack: Walnuts and dried apricots.
- Dinner: Baked cod with sweet potatoes and green beans.

Friday

- Breakfast: Oatmeal pancakes with banana and berries.
- Snack: Carrots and hummus.
- Lunch: Quinoa salad with vegetables, feta, and olives.
- Snack: Greek yogurt with nuts and honey.
- Dinner: Baked chicken breast with millet and vegetables.

Saturday

- Breakfast: Fried eggs with whole grain toast and avocado.
- Snack: Smoothie with plant protein, berries, and spinach.
- Lunch: Pumpkin soup with pumpkin seeds and whole grain bread.
- Snack: Cashews and dried apricots.
- Dinner: Grilled steak with vegetables and arugula salad.

Sunday

- Breakfast: Oatmeal with almonds, chia seeds, and fresh fruits.
- Snack: Celery sticks with peanut butter.
- Lunch: Whole grain wraps with vegetables, hummus, and chicken.

- Snack: Greek yogurt with honey and nuts.
- Dinner: Baked salmon with quinoa and broccoli.

Option 2: Vegetarian

Monday

- Breakfast: Oatmeal with fruits, nuts, and flaxseed.
- Snack: Natural yogurt with honey and berries.
- Lunch: Chickpea salad with avocado, tomatoes, and olive oil.
- Snack: Carrots and hummus.
- Dinner: Stir-fry with tofu, vegetables, and brown rice.

Tuesday

- Breakfast: Scrambled eggs with vegetables and whole grain bread.
- Snack: Nuts and dried fruits.
- Lunch: Lentil soup with vegetables.
- Snack: Celery sticks with peanut butter.
- Dinner: Baked zucchini with quinoa and vegetables.

Wednesday

- Breakfast: Smoothie with kale, banana, berries, and almond milk.
- Snack: Chia seeds with yogurt and honey.
- Lunch: Whole grain pasta with tomato sauce, tofu, and spinach.
- Snack: Apple with almond butter.
- Dinner: Bean salad with egg, olives, and vegetables.

Thursday

- Breakfast: Toast with avocado and poached egg.
- Snack: Smoothie with plant protein, spinach, and berries.
- Lunch: Stir-fry with tempeh, vegetables, and brown rice.
- Snack: Walnuts and dried apricots.
- Dinner: Baked eggplant with sweet potatoes and green beans.

Friday

- Breakfast: Oatmeal pancakes with banana and berries.
- Snack: Carrots and hummus.
- Lunch: Quinoa salad with vegetables, feta, and olives.
- Snack: Greek yogurt with nuts and honey.

- Dinner: Baked tofu with millet and vegetables.

Saturday

- Breakfast: Fried eggs with whole grain toast and avocado.
- Snack: Smoothie with plant protein, berries, and spinach.
- Lunch: Pumpkin soup with pumpkin seeds and whole grain bread.
- Snack: Cashews and dried apricots.
- Dinner: Grilled vegetables with basmati rice and arugula salad.

Sunday

- Breakfast: Oatmeal with almonds, chia seeds, and fresh fruits.
- Snack: Celery sticks with peanut butter.
- Lunch: Whole grain wraps with vegetables, hummus, and tempeh.
- Snack: Greek yogurt with honey and nuts.
- Dinner: Baked vegetables with quinoa and broccoli.

Option 3: Low-Carb Diet

Monday

- Breakfast: Omelet with vegetables and feta cheese.
- Snack: Hard-boiled eggs.
- Lunch: Chicken salad with avocado, tomatoes, and olive oil.
- Snack: Celery sticks with peanut butter.
- Dinner: Grilled salmon with broccoli and cauliflower.

Tuesday

- Breakfast: Greek yogurt with nuts and berries.
- Snack: Cucumber slices with hummus.
- Lunch: Broccoli cream soup with cheddar cheese.
- Snack: Almonds.
- Dinner: Baked chicken breast with asparagus and green beans.

Wednesday

- Breakfast: Smoothie with kale, avocado, plant protein, and almond milk.
- Snack: Carrots with guacamole.
- Lunch: Tuna salad with egg, olives, and vegetables.
- Snack: Natural yogurt with honey.
- Dinner: Baked cod with Brussels sprouts and roasted vegetables.

Thursday

- Breakfast: Soft-boiled eggs with avocado and tomato.
- Snack: Walnuts.
- Lunch: Stir-fry with tofu, vegetables, and cashews.
- Snack: Celery sticks with almond butter.
- Dinner: Baked eggplant with feta and spinach.

Friday

- Breakfast: Spinach and egg pancakes.
- Snack: Berries with Greek yogurt.
- Lunch: Shrimp salad with avocado, tomatoes, and olive oil.
- Snack: Chia seeds with coconut milk.
- Dinner: Grilled steak with arugula and tomato salad.

Saturday

- Breakfast: Eggs Benedict with hollandaise sauce.
- Snack: Carrot slices with hummus.
- Lunch: Pumpkin cream soup with pumpkin seeds.
- Snack: Cashews.
- Dinner: Grilled cod with kale salad.

Sunday

- Breakfast: Omelet with mushrooms, spinach, and cheddar cheese.

- Snack: Apple with peanut butter.
- Lunch: Whole grain wraps with vegetables, hummus, and chicken.
- Snack: Greek yogurt with honey and nuts.
- Dinner: Baked salmon with quinoa and broccoli.

Option 4: Mediterranean Diet

Monday

- Breakfast: Greek yogurt with honey, nuts, and fruits.
- Snack: Olives and feta cheese.
- Lunch: Greek salad with chicken, tomatoes, cucumber, olives, and feta.
- Snack: Celery sticks with hummus.
- Dinner: Grilled salmon with roasted vegetables and quinoa.

Tuesday

- Breakfast: Omelet with vegetables, feta cheese, and olives.
- Snack: A handful of almonds.
- Lunch: Chickpea soup with vegetables and tomatoes.
- Snack: Carrot slices with hummus.

- Dinner: Tuna salad with avocado, egg, olives, and vegetables.

Wednesday

- Breakfast: Smoothie with kale, banana, berries, and almond milk.
- Snack: Celery sticks with peanut butter.
- Lunch: Whole grain pasta with tomato sauce, olives, capers, and basil.
- Snack: Apple with nuts.
- Dinner: Baked cod with sweet potatoes and arugula salad.

Thursday

- Breakfast: Fried eggs with avocado and whole grain toast.
- Snack: Greek yogurt with honey and nuts.
- Lunch: Stir-fry with tofu, vegetables, and cashews.
- Snack: Olives and feta cheese.
- Dinner: Baked eggplant with tomatoes, mozzarella, and basil.

Friday

- Breakfast: Oatmeal with fruits, nuts, and honey.

- Snack: A handful of cashews.
- Lunch: Grilled vegetable salad with feta and quinoa.
- Snack: Cucumber slices with hummus.
- Dinner: Grilled steak with arugula and tomato salad.

Saturday

- Breakfast: Eggs Benedict with whole grain toast.
- Snack: Carrot slices with hummus.
- Lunch: Minestrone soup with beans and vegetables.
- Snack: A handful of almonds.
- Dinner: Grilled cod with kale salad.

Sunday

- Breakfast: Omelet with vegetables, feta cheese, and olives.
- Snack: Apple with peanut butter.
- Lunch: Whole grain wraps with vegetables, hummus, and chicken.
- Snack: Greek yogurt with honey and nuts.
- Dinner: Baked salmon with quinoa and broccoli.

Option 5: Vegan Diet

Monday

- Breakfast: Oatmeal with fruits, nuts, and flaxseed.

- Snack: Coconut yogurt with honey and berries.
- Lunch: Chickpea salad with avocado, tomatoes, and olive oil.
- Snack: Carrots and hummus.
- Dinner: Stir-fry with tofu, vegetables, and brown rice.

Tuesday

- Breakfast: Smoothie with kale, banana, berries, and almond milk.
- Snack: Chia seeds with coconut yogurt and honey.
- Lunch: Lentil soup with vegetables.
- Snack: Celery sticks with peanut butter.
- Dinner: Baked zucchini with quinoa and vegetables.

Wednesday

- Breakfast: Toast with avocado and chia seeds.
- Snack: Nuts and dried fruits.
- Lunch: Whole grain pasta with tomato sauce, tofu, and spinach.
- Snack: Apple with almond butter.
- Dinner: Bean salad with avocado, olives, and vegetables.

Thursday

- Breakfast: Tofu scramble with vegetables and whole grain bread.
- Snack: Smoothie with plant protein, spinach, and berries.
- Lunch: Stir-fry with tempeh, vegetables, and brown rice.
- Snack: Walnuts and dried apricots.
- Dinner: Baked eggplant with sweet potatoes and green beans.

Friday

- Breakfast: Oatmeal pancakes with banana and berries.
- Snack: Carrots and hummus.
- Lunch: Quinoa salad with vegetables, tofu, and olives.
- Snack: Coconut yogurt with nuts and honey.
- Dinner: Baked tofu with millet and vegetables.

Saturday

- Breakfast: Tofu scramble with vegetables.
- Snack: Smoothie with plant protein, berries, and spinach.
- Lunch: Pumpkin soup with pumpkin seeds and whole grain bread.
- Snack: Cashews and dried apricots.
- Dinner: Grilled vegetables with basmati rice and arugula salad.

Sunday

- Breakfast: Oatmeal with almonds, chia seeds, and fresh fruits.
- Snack: Celery sticks with peanut butter.
- Lunch: Whole grain wraps with vegetables, hummus, and tempeh.

- Snack: Coconut yogurt with honey and nuts.
- Dinner: Baked vegetables with quinoa and broccoli.

A healthy diet during menopause should be balanced, varied, and rich in nutrients. Superfoods such as soy, flaxseed, fatty fish, cruciferous vegetables, nuts, berries, avocado, and olive oil can support hormonal health and alleviate menopausal symptoms. The sample meal plans for the week present various dietary options that can be adjusted to individual needs and preferences. Remember that regular consumption of healthy meals, proper hydration, and avoiding processed foods are key elements of effective weight and health management during menopause.

Chapter 4: Physical Exercise

Physical exercise is crucial for maintaining health, fitness, and managing weight during menopause. Regular physical activity helps reduce stress, improve sleep quality, increase muscle mass, and enhance cardiovascular health. In this chapter, we will discuss different types of exercises and provide three workout plans tailored to various skill levels and preferences.

Types of Exercises

1. Aerobic Exercises

Aerobic exercises, also known as cardio, increase the heart rate and improve cardiovascular endurance. Examples of aerobic exercises include walking, running, cycling, swimming, and dancing.

Benefits:

- Improved heart and circulatory health
- Increased endurance
- Calorie burning
- Stress reduction

Plan 1: Walking

Beginner:

- Day 1: 20 minutes of walking at a moderate pace
- Day 2: 20 minutes of walking at a moderate pace
- Day 3: Rest
- Day 4: 25 minutes of walking at a moderate pace
- Day 5: 20 minutes of walking at a brisk pace
- Day 6: 30 minutes of walking at a moderate pace
- Day 7: Rest

Intermediate:

- Day 1: 30 minutes of walking at a brisk pace
- Day 2: 25 minutes of walking at a moderate pace
- Day 3: 30 minutes of walking at a brisk pace
- Day 4: Rest
- Day 5: 35 minutes of walking at a moderate pace

- Day 6: 30 minutes of walking at a brisk pace
- Day 7: 40 minutes of walking at a moderate pace

Advanced:

- Day 1: 45 minutes of walking at a brisk pace
- Day 2: 40 minutes of walking at a moderate pace
- Day 3: 45 minutes of walking at a brisk pace
- Day 4: 50 minutes of walking at a moderate pace
- Day 5: 45 minutes of walking at a brisk pace
- Day 6: 60 minutes of walking at a moderate pace
- Day 7: Rest

Plan 2: Running

Beginner:

- Day 1: 10 minutes of walk-jog intervals (30 seconds running, 2 minutes walking)
- Day 2: Rest
- Day 3: 12 minutes of walk-jog intervals (45 seconds running, 2 minutes walking)

- Day 4: Rest

- Day 5: 15 minutes of walk-jog intervals (60 seconds running, 2 minutes walking)

- Day 6: Rest

- Day 7: 18 minutes of walk-jog intervals (60 seconds running, 90 seconds walking)

Intermediate:

- Day 1: 20 minutes of running (2 minutes running, 1 minute walking)

- Day 2: Rest

- Day 3: 25 minutes of running (3 minutes running, 1 minute walking)

- Day 4: Rest

- Day 5: 30 minutes of running (4 minutes running, 1 minute walking)

- Day 6: Rest

- Day 7: 35 minutes of running (5 minutes running, 1 minute walking)

Advanced:

- Day 1: 40 minutes of continuous running

- Day 2: Rest

- Day 3: 45 minutes of continuous running
- Day 4: Rest
- Day 5: 50 minutes of continuous running
- Day 6: Rest
- Day 7: 60 minutes of continuous running

Plan 3: Cycling

Beginner:

Day 1: 20 minutes of cycling at a moderate pace

Day 2: Rest

Day 3: 25 minutes of cycling at a moderate pace

Day 4: Rest

Day 5: 30 minutes of cycling at a moderate pace

Day 6: Rest

Day 7: 35 minutes of cycling at a moderate pace

Intermediate:

- Day 1: 40 minutes of cycling at a fast pace

- Day 2: Rest

- Day 3: 45 minutes of cycling at a moderate pace

- Day 4: Rest

- Day 5: 50 minutes of cycling at a fast pace

- Day 6: Rest

- Day 7: 55 minutes of cycling at a moderate pace

Advanced:

- Day 1: 60 minutes of cycling at a fast pace

- Day 2: Rest

- Day 3: 70 minutes of cycling at a moderate pace

- Day 4: Rest

- Day 5: 80 minutes of cycling at a fast pace

- Day 6: Rest

- Day 7: 90 minutes of cycling at a moderate pace

2. Strength Training

Strength training helps build muscle mass, strengthen bones, and improve metabolism. Examples of strength exercises include weightlifting, resistance band exercises, and bodyweight training.

Benefits:

- Increased muscle mass
- Bone strengthening
- Boosted metabolism
- Improved posture

Strength Training Plans:

Plan 1: Bodyweight Training

Beginner:

- Squats: 3 sets of 10 reps
- Knee push-ups: 3 sets of 8 reps
- Plank: 3 sets of 20 seconds
- Lunges: 3 sets of 8 reps per leg
- Rest between sets: 60 seconds

Intermediate:

- Squats: 3 sets of 15 reps
- Push-ups: 3 sets of 10 reps
- Plank: 3 sets of 30 seconds
- Lunges: 3 sets of 12 reps per leg
- Rest between sets: 45 seconds

Advanced:

- Single-leg squats: 3 sets of 8 reps per leg
- Push-ups: 3 sets of 15 reps
- Plank with leg lift: 3 sets of 40 seconds
- Walking lunges: 3 sets of 20 reps per leg
- Rest between sets: 30 seconds

Plan 2: Weight Training

Beginner:

- Dumbbell squats: 3 sets of 10 reps
- Dumbbell bench press: 3 sets of 10 reps

- Dumbbell deadlift: 3 sets of 8 reps
- Bent-over dumbbell rows: 3 sets of 10 reps
- Rest between sets: 60 seconds

Intermediate:

- Dumbbell squats: 3 sets of 15 reps
- Dumbbell bench press: 3 sets of 12 reps
- Dumbbell deadlift: 3 sets of 10 reps
- Bent-over dumbbell rows: 3 sets of 12 reps
- Rest between sets: 45 seconds

Advanced:

- Barbell squats: 3 sets of 10 reps
- Barbell bench press: 3 sets of 8 reps
- Deadlift: 3 sets of 8 reps
- Bent-over barbell rows: 3 sets of 10 reps
- Rest between sets: 30 seconds
- Plan 3: Resistance Band Training

Beginner:

- Resistance band squats: 3 sets of 10 reps

- Resistance band chest press: 3 sets of 10 reps

- Resistance band deadlift: 3 sets of 8 reps

- Resistance band rows: 3 sets of 10 reps

- Rest between sets: 60 seconds

Intermediate:

- Resistance band squats: 3 sets of 15 reps

- Resistance band chest press: 3 sets of 12 reps

- Resistance band deadlift: 3 sets of 10 reps

- Resistance band rows: 3 sets of 12 reps

- Rest between sets: 45 seconds

Advanced:

- Resistance band squats: 3 sets of 20 reps

- Resistance band chest press: 3 sets of 15 reps

- Resistance band deadlift: 3 sets of 12 reps

- Resistance band rows: 3 sets of 15 reps

- Rest between sets: 30 seconds

Stretching and mobility exercises improve flexibility, balance, and reduce muscle tension. Examples include yoga, Pilates, and dynamic stretching.

Benefits:

- Improved flexibility
- Reduced injury risk
- Muscle tension reduction
- Improved posture
- Stretching and Mobility Plans:

Plan 1: Yoga

Beginner:

- Day 1: 20 minutes of yoga (basic poses: Tadasana, Bhujangasana, Balasana)
- Day 2: Rest
- Day 3: 20 minutes of yoga (basic poses: Virabhadrasana I, Uttanasana, Shavasana)
- Day 4: Rest
- Day 5: 20 minutes of yoga (basic poses: Adho Mukha Svanasana, Setu Bandhasana, Sukhasana)
- Day 6: Rest
- Day 7: 20 minutes of yoga (basic poses: Vrksasana, Dandasana, Supta Baddha Konasana)

Intermediate:

- Day 1: 30 minutes of yoga (poses: Trikonasana, Parsvakonasana, Salabhasana)
- Day 2: Rest
- Day 3: 30 minutes of yoga (poses: Utkatasana, Ardha Chandrasana, Savasana)
- Day 4: Rest
- Day 5: 30 minutes of yoga (poses: Bakasana, Navasana, Viparita Karani)
- Day 6: Rest

- Day 7: 30 minutes of yoga (poses: Halasana, Sarvangasana, Shavasana)

Advanced:

- Day 1: 45 minutes of yoga (poses: Hanumanasana, Kakasana, Shavasana)
- Day 2: Rest
- Day 3: 45 minutes of yoga (poses: Pincha Mayurasana, Kapotasana, Shavasana)
- Day 4: Rest
- Day 5: 45 minutes of yoga (poses: Eka Pada Rajakapotasana, Mayurasana, Shavasana)
- Day 6: Rest
- Day 7: 45 minutes of yoga (poses: Adho Mukha Vrksasana, Sirsasana, Shavasana)

Plan 2: Pilates

Beginner:

- Day 1: 20 minutes of Pilates (basic exercises: The Hundred, Roll-Up, Leg Circles)
- Day 2: Rest
- Day 3: 20 minutes of Pilates (basic exercises: Single-Leg Stretch,

- Double-Leg Stretch, Spine Stretch)
- Day 4: Rest
- Day 5: 20 minutes of Pilates (basic exercises: Saw, Pelvic Curl, Leg Pull Front)
- Day 6: Rest
- Day 7: 20 minutes of Pilates (basic exercises: Swimming, Side Kick, Seal)

Intermediate:

- Day 1: 30 minutes of Pilates (exercises: The Hundred, Roll-Up, Single Straight Leg Stretch)
- Day 2: Rest
- Day 3: 30 minutes of Pilates (exercises: Double-Leg Stretch, Criss-Cross, Spine Stretch Forward)
- Day 4: Rest
- Day 5: 30 minutes of Pilates (exercises: Open Leg Rocker, Corkscrew, Saw)
- Day 6: Rest
- Day 7: 30 minutes of Pilates (exercises: Swimming, Side Bend, Seal)

Advanced:

- Day 1: 45 minutes of Pilates (exercises: The Hundred, Roll-Over, Scissors)

- Day 2: Rest

- Day 3: 45 minutes of Pilates (exercises: Double-Leg Stretch, Teaser, Spine Twist)

- Day 4: Rest

- Day 5: 45 minutes of Pilates (exercises: Boomerang, Jackknife, Bicycle)

- Day 6: Rest

- Day 7: 45 minutes of Pilates (exercises: Side Kick Series, Leg Pull Front, Push-Up)

Plan 3: Dynamic Stretching

Beginner:

- Day 1: 10 minutes of dynamic stretching (exercises: Arm Circles, Leg Swings, Hip Circles)

- Day 2: Rest

- Day 3: 10 minutes of dynamic stretching (exercises: Walking Lunges, High Knees, Torso Twists)

- Day 4: Rest

- Day 5: 10 minutes of dynamic stretching (exercises: Arm Circles, Leg Swings, Hip Circles)

- Day 6: Rest

- Day 7: 10 minutes of dynamic stretching (exercises: Walking Lunges, High Knees, Torso Twists)

Intermediate:

- Day 1: 15 minutes of dynamic stretching (exercises: Arm Circles, Leg Swings, Hip Circles, Walking Lunges)

- Day 2: Rest

- Day 3: 15 minutes of dynamic stretching (exercises: High Knees, Torso Twists, Lateral Lunges)

- Day 4: Rest

- Day 5: 15 minutes of dynamic stretching (exercises: Arm Circles, Leg Swings, Hip Circles, Walking Lunges)

- Day 6: Rest

- Day 7: 15 minutes of dynamic stretching (exercises: High Knees, Torso Twists, Lateral Lunges)

Advanced:

- Day 1: 20 minutes of dynamic stretching (exercises: Arm

Circles, Leg Swings, Hip Circles, Walking Lunges, High Knees)

- Day 2: Rest
- Day 3: 20 minutes of dynamic stretching (exercises: Torso Twists, Lateral Lunges, Butt Kicks, Skipping)
- Day 4: Rest
- Day 5: 20 minutes of dynamic stretching (exercises: Arm Circles, Leg Swings, Hip Circles, Walking Lunges, High Knees)
- Day 6: Rest
- Day 7: 20 minutes of dynamic stretching (exercises: Torso Twists, Lateral Lunges, Butt Kicks, Skipping)

Getting Started

If you are just starting out, it is crucial to gradually introduce exercises into your daily routine. Begin with short sessions that you can gradually extend. Always remember to warm up before exercises and cool down after completing them. Listen to your body and avoid overexerting yourself in the beginning.

Basic Guidelines:

- **Warm-Up:** Always start with a warm-up to prepare your muscles and joints for exertion. This can be 5-10 minutes of light cardio, such as marching in place, jumping rope, or dynamic stretching.

- **Cool Down:** After completing exercises, perform 5-10 minutes of gentle walking or light stretching to help your body return to a resting state.

- **Gradual Increase in Intensity:** Begin with low intensity and gradually increase the duration and intensity of your workouts to avoid injury.

- **Variety:** Vary your workouts to engage different muscle groups and maintain motivation.

- **Rest:** Give yourself time to recover, especially if you are just starting out or increasing the intensity of your workouts.

Regular physical activity is essential for maintaining health and managing weight during menopause. By choosing a variety of exercises, such as aerobic exercises, strength training, and stretching and mobility, you can improve your fitness, increase muscle mass, reduce stress, and enhance overall well-being. The workout plans provided in this chapter offer different levels of intensity and types of exercises that can be tailored to your individual preferences and abilities. Remember to always listen to your body and gradually increase workout intensity to avoid injury and achieve the best results.

Chapter 5: Lifestyle

Lifestyle plays a crucial role in managing weight and health during menopause. It includes stress management, sleep quality, and emotional support. In this chapter, we will discuss these aspects in detail and provide specific tips to improve your lifestyle.

Stress Management

Stress is a common issue during menopause, and effective stress management is essential for maintaining health and quality of life.

Relaxation Techniques

Meditation: Regular meditation can help reduce stress, improve concentration, and enhance overall well-being. Mindfulness meditation, which focuses on being present in the moment, can be particularly effective.

- **How to start:** Find a quiet place, sit comfortably, close your eyes, and focus on your breath. When thoughts wander, gently redirect them to your breath. Start with 5-10 minutes daily and gradually increase the time.

Yoga: Yoga combines physical exercises, breathing techniques, and meditation, which help reduce stress and improve flexibility and strength.

- **How to start:** Begin with simple poses (asanas) and breathing techniques (pranayama). Many free online resources, such as YouTube videos, offer yoga sessions for beginners.

Deep Breathing: Simple deep breathing techniques can help reduce stress immediately.

- **How to start:** Try diaphragmatic breathing – take a deep breath through your nose, letting your abdomen rise, then exhale slowly through your mouth.

Progressive Muscle Relaxation: This technique involves gradually tensing and relaxing different muscle groups, which helps reduce tension and stress.

- **How to start:** Start from your feet, tense muscles for 5 seconds, then relax. Move to the next muscle group until you reach your head.

Recreational Activities

- **Hobbies:** Engaging in hobbies like reading, gardening, painting, or crafting can be an excellent way to relax and de-stress.

- **Outdoor Time:** Spending time outdoors, such as walking in the park, can improve your mood and reduce stress levels.

- **Music:** Listening to your favorite music can have a relaxing effect and improve your mood.

Sleep and Its Importance

Sleep problems are a common symptom of menopause. Good quality sleep is crucial for physical and mental health. Here's how to improve sleep quality:

Creating the Right Sleep Environment

- **Regular Sleep Schedule:** Try to go to bed and wake up at the same time every day, even on weekends.

- **Bedroom Environment:** Ensure your bedroom is dark, quiet, and cool. Invest in a comfortable mattress and pillows.

- **Limiting Blue Light Exposure:** Avoid using electronic devices like TVs, computers, and smartphones at least an hour before bedtime.

Preparing for Sleep

- **Bedtime Rituals:** Create a routine that helps you relax before bed. This could be a warm bath, reading a book, or listening to calm music.

- **Avoid Heavy Meals and Caffeine:** Have your last meal at least 2-3 hours before sleep. Avoid caffeine and alcohol several hours before bedtime as they can disrupt sleep.

- **Relaxation Techniques:** Meditate, practice deep breathing, or progressive muscle relaxation before bed to help you fall asleep.

Tracking Sleep

- **Sleep Journal:** Keep a sleep journal to record sleep hours, nighttime awakenings, and sleep quality. This will help identify patterns and potential problems.

Emotional Support

Emotional support is key in managing stress and emotions during menopause. Here's how to get it:

Family and Friends

- **Open Conversations:** Talk to loved ones about your feelings and experiences. Emotional support from family and friends can be extremely helpful.

- **Partner Support:** If you have a partner, discuss menopause together to understand and support each other.

Support Groups

- **Local Support Groups:** Join local support groups for

women going through menopause. Sharing experiences with others can be inspiring and comforting.

- **Online Groups:** There are many online support groups where you can share your experiences, ask questions, and get support from other women going through menopause.

Professional Help

Individual Therapy: Consulting a psychologist or therapist can help in coping with emotions and stress.

Family Counseling: Family therapy can aid in communication and mutual support within the family.

Lifestyle and Dietary Changes

Diet

- **Balanced Diet:** Eat a diet rich in protein, healthy fats, fiber, and complex carbohydrates.

- **Superfoods:** Include superfoods like berries, nuts, avocado, flaxseeds, and fatty fish in your diet, which are rich in essential nutrients.

- **Avoid Processed Foods:** Limit the intake of processed foods, simple sugars, and trans fats.

- **Regular Meals:** Eat regular meals to maintain steady energy levels and avoid hunger pangs.

Physical Activity

- **Regular Exercise:** Exercise regularly, combining strength training, aerobic activities, and stretching. Regular exercise helps maintain a healthy weight, improve fitness, and reduce stress.

- **Daily Activity:** Try to stay active every day. Even short walks can provide health benefits.

- **Choose Enjoyable Activities:** Exercise should be enjoyable, not a chore. Choose activities you like, such as dancing, swimming, or cycling.

Avoiding Addictions

- **Limiting Alcohol:** Alcohol can exacerbate menopausal symptoms and affect sleep and weight. Limit alcohol consumption.

- **Quitting Smoking:** Smoking increases the risk of many diseases, including heart disease and osteoporosis. Quitting smoking provides health benefits at any age.

Managing lifestyle during menopause is crucial for maintaining health and quality of life. Relaxation techniques, ensuring good sleep quality, emotional support, a healthy diet, and regular physical activity can significantly improve well-being and help cope with menopausal symptoms. Regularly monitoring progress and making lifestyle changes can bring long-term health benefits.

Chapter 6: Tracking Progress

Tracking progress during menopause is a key element of effective health and weight management. Keeping a health journal that includes diet, exercise, symptom tracking, and result measurement can significantly help maintain motivation and assess the effectiveness of your actions.

Health Journal

1. Diet Logging

Keeping a diet journal can help identify eating habits, control calorie and macronutrient intake, and monitor how different foods affect menopausal symptoms.

- **Daily Records:** Note everything you eat and drink each day, including snacks and beverages. Records can include meal times, quantities, and types of food consumed.
- **Macronutrients:** Pay attention to the intake of proteins, fats, and carbohydrates. Aim to maintain a balanced diet rich in protein, healthy fats, and fiber.

- **Hydration:** Record the amount of water and other beverages consumed. Staying properly hydrated is crucial for health.

- **Reactions to Foods:** Note how you feel after eating different foods. This helps identify foods that may exacerbate menopausal symptoms or cause discomfort.

2. Exercise Monitoring

Regular physical activity is crucial for health and weight management. Keeping an exercise journal helps track progress and motivates continued workouts.

- **Types of Exercises:** Note the type of physical activity (e.g., running, walking, yoga, strength training).

- **Duration and Intensity:** Record the duration of each workout and its intensity. You can use a scale from 1 to 10 to rate the effort level.

- **Frequency:** Note how often you exercise. Regularity is key to maintaining health and fitness.

- **Progress:** Record achievements such as kilometers run, weights lifted, or increased flexibility. Tracking progress can be very motivating.

3. Symptom Tracking

Menopause is associated with many symptoms that can affect daily life. Tracking symptoms helps understand how different factors influence your well-being and how to manage symptoms effectively.

- **Daily Symptom Records:** Record symptoms that occur each day, such as hot flashes, night sweats, mood swings, fatigue, or insomnia.
- **Symptom Severity:** Rate the severity of symptoms on a scale from 1 to 10. This helps identify patterns and triggers.
- **Triggers:** Note situations, foods, or other factors that may exacerbate menopausal symptoms.
- **Treatments and Interventions:** Record any treatments or interventions you use and their effectiveness.

4. Measuring Results

Regular monitoring of results allows you to track changes in body weight, body composition, and overall health.

- **Body Weight:** Weigh yourself regularly, preferably at the same time of day, to track changes in weight.

- **Body Measurements:** Measure the circumference of your waist, hips, thighs, and arms to monitor changes in body composition.

- **Body Fat Percentage:** If you have access to devices that measure body fat percentage, check these values regularly.

- **Strength and Fitness:** Note changes in physical strength and fitness, such as increased weights lifted during strength training or improved endurance during aerobic exercises.

Goals and Motivation

1. Setting Realistic Goals

Goals should be specific, measurable, achievable, realistic, and time-bound (SMART). Setting such goals helps track progress and maintain motivation.

- **Specific:** Define exactly what you want to achieve (e.g., "I want to lose 5 kg in 3 months").

- **Measurable:** Establish how you will measure progress (e.g., "I will weigh myself once a week and measure body circumferences every month").

- **Achievable:** Ensure goals are realistic and achievable (e.g., "I will exercise for 30 minutes a day, 5 days a week").

- **Realistic:** Ensure goals are appropriate for your situation and capabilities (e.g., "I will stick to a diet rich in protein and vegetables").

- **Time-bound:** Specify the timeframe for achieving the goal (e.g., "I want to lose 5 kg in 3 months").

2. Small Steps

Break down large goals into smaller, more manageable steps. This helps maintain motivation and provides a sense of accomplishment at each stage.

- **Daily Goals:** Small changes that can be made daily, e.g., "Today, I will drink more water" or "Today, I will take a 10-minute walk".

- **Weekly Goals:** Goals for each week, e.g., "This week, I will eat five servings of vegetables daily" or "This week, I will complete three workout sessions".

- **Monthly Goals:** Larger goals achievable within a month, e.g., "This month, I will lose 2 kg" or "This month, I will increase the intensity of my workouts".

3. Rewards

Rewarding yourself for achieving goals can boost motivation. It is important that rewards are healthy and do not conflict with your health goals.

- **Small Rewards:** Treat yourself for small achievements, e.g., a new book, a movie night, or a relaxing bath.
- **Larger Rewards:** For bigger achievements, e.g., a weekend getaway, new sportswear, or a massage.

4. Support from Loved Ones

Sharing your goals with loved ones and asking for support can help maintain motivation and accountability.

- **Family and Friends:** Inform loved ones about your goals and ask for their support. They can help you stick to your plan and motivate you during difficult moments.

- **Support Groups:** Join online or local support groups where you can share experiences and receive support from other women going through menopause.
- **Professionals:** Seek help from a dietitian, personal trainer, or therapist who can assist in setting goals, tracking progress, and maintaining motivation.

Tracking progress with a health journal that includes diet, exercise, symptom tracking, and result measurement is key to effective health and weight management during menopause. Setting realistic goals, breaking them into small steps, rewarding yourself for achievements, and seeking support from loved ones are effective strategies to help maintain motivation and achieve success. Regular monitoring of progress allows you to assess the effectiveness of your actions and make necessary changes, leading to better health and well-being.

Chapter 7: Medical Support

When to Consult a Doctor

Certain symptoms and health issues require consultation with a doctor:

- **Intensifying Menopausal Symptoms:** If symptoms such as hot flashes, night sweats, mood swings, or sleep problems are severe enough to impact your quality of life, you should consult a doctor.

- **Irregular or Unusual Bleeding:** Any unusual bleeding after menopause should be discussed with a doctor as it may indicate health issues such as polyps, endometrial hyperplasia, or endometrial cancer.

- **Severe Headaches:** If you experience new or worsening headaches that are particularly intense or frequent, a consultation with a neurologist may be necessary.

- **Sudden Weight Gain:** Significant and rapid weight gain without an obvious cause may indicate hormonal problems such as thyroid disorders.

- **Breast Changes:** Any changes in the breasts, such as lumps, changes in shape, or discharge from the nipples, should be immediately evaluated by a doctor.

- **Heart Problems:** Hormonal changes can increase the risk of heart disease. Symptoms such as chest pain,

- shortness of breath, dizziness, and palpitations require immediate medical consultation.

Treatment Options

There are many ways to treat menopausal symptoms and support weight loss, which can be tailored to each woman's individual needs:

Hormone Replacement Therapy (HRT)

- **Estrogen Replacement Therapy (ERT):** Recommended for women who have had a hysterectomy (removal of the uterus). It can alleviate menopausal symptoms such as hot flashes, vaginal dryness, and mood swings.

- **Estrogen-Progestogen Therapy (EPT):** Used for women who have a uterus. The combination of estrogen and progestogen reduces the risk of endometrial cancer, which can be increased by estrogen alone. It also helps alleviate menopausal symptoms.

- **Bioidentical Hormone Therapy:** These hormones are chemically identical to those produced by the human body. They can be used in creams, patches, tablets, or implants.

Prescription Medications

- **Antidepressants:** Some antidepressants, such as selective serotonin reuptake inhibitors (SSRIs) and serotonin-norepinephrine reuptake inhibitors (SNRIs), can help alleviate hot flashes and mood swings.

- **Blood Pressure Medications:** Medications such as clonidine can be effective in reducing the frequency and severity of hot flashes.

- **Gabapentin:** An anticonvulsant that can help relieve hot flashes and improve sleep.

- **Osteoporosis Treatments:** Bisphosphonates, denosumab, raloxifene, and hormone therapies can be used to prevent bone loss and treat osteoporosis.

Dietary Supplements

- **Calcium and Vitamin D:** Essential for bone health. Supplementation may be particularly important for women at risk of osteoporosis.

- **Magnesium:** Helps combat fatigue, muscle cramps, and insomnia.

- **Omega-3 Fatty Acids:** Can support heart and brain health and alleviate symptoms of depression.

- **Phytoestrogens:** Found in plants like soy and flaxseed, they can help alleviate menopausal symptoms.

Alternative and Complementary Therapies

- **Acupuncture:** Can help relieve hot flashes, pain, and stress.
- **Herbal Medicine:** Herbs such as black cohosh, St. John's wort, and hops can be used to alleviate menopausal symptoms. However, it is important to consult a doctor before starting any herbal therapy.
- **Homeopathy:** Some women report benefits from homeopathic treatment, although scientific evidence of its effectiveness is limited.
- **Meditation and Relaxation Techniques:** Can help manage stress and improve overall well-being.

Lifestyle and Dietary Changes

- **Healthy Diet:** Eating a balanced diet rich in protein, healthy fats, fiber, and complex carbohydrates can help manage weight and menopausal symptoms.
- **Regular Physical Activity:** Aerobic exercises, strength training, and stretching can improve fitness, increase muscle mass, and reduce menopausal symptoms.

- **Relaxation Techniques:** Yoga, tai chi, meditation, and deep breathing can help reduce stress and improve sleep quality.
- **Avoiding Triggers:** Such as caffeine, alcohol, spicy foods, and stress, which can exacerbate menopausal symptoms.

Considerations for Treatment

Every woman experiences menopause differently, so it is important to tailor the treatment plan individually. Some women may need a combination of different methods to effectively manage symptoms and improve quality of life. Regular consultations with a doctor are essential to monitor health and adjust the treatment plan as needed.

Medical support during menopause can include a wide range of methods, from pharmacotherapy to lifestyle changes and alternative therapies. The key is to find the right methods that will be effective for the individual. Regular consultations with a doctor, a healthy diet, physical activity, and relaxation techniques can significantly improve the quality of life during this important period.

Chapter 8: Success Stories

Case Studies

Mary, 52 years old

Mary noticed that she began gaining weight after menopause, even though her eating habits hadn't changed significantly. After consulting with her doctor, she learned that the drop in estrogen levels affected her metabolism and fat distribution. She decided to make changes to her lifestyle.

Mary adopted a diet rich in phytoestrogens, such as soy, flaxseed, and whole grain products. Additionally, she reduced the amount of processed foods and sugar in her diet. She also started exercising regularly, choosing mainly walking, yoga, and light strength training.

After a few months, Mary noticed a significant improvement in her well-being. She managed to lose 7 kg, and her menopausal symptoms, such as hot flashes and mood swings, significantly decreased. Mary continues her healthy lifestyle and enjoys better health.

Anna, 49 years old

Anna noticed that her weight started to increase, even though her eating habits and level of physical activity remained the same. Understanding that metabolic changes associated with menopause might be responsible for the weight gain, Anna decided to make some key changes.

Anna began regular strength training, which helped her increase muscle mass and speed up her metabolism. She incorporated more protein, healthy fats, and fiber into her diet. Additionally, she started drinking more water and reduced alcohol consumption.

After a few months of regular exercise and a healthy diet, Anna lost 10 kg and felt more energetic. Her physical condition improved significantly, and she gained confidence and satisfaction with life.

Patricia, 55 years old

Patricia had difficulty falling asleep and often woke up at night.

She felt tired and started eating more unhealthy snacks, which led to weight gain. She decided to make changes to improve her sleep quality and manage her weight.

Patricia began practicing relaxation techniques, such as meditation and yoga, which helped improve her sleep quality and reduce stress. She also changed her eating habits by incorporating more vegetables, fruits, and whole grain products into her diet. She avoided late-night snacks and tried to eat regular meals.

After a few months, Patricia noticed a significant improvement in her sleep quality. She managed to lose 5 kg, and her well-being improved significantly. Thanks to the changes she made, Patricia now feels more rested and healthy.

Cynthia, 50 years old

Cynthia started with a beginner's training program and gradually increased the intensity of her exercises. She also decided to change her eating habits to better suit her body's needs.

Cynthia incorporated more protein, healthy fats, and fiber into her diet. She exercised regularly, choosing activities she enjoyed, such as walking, yoga, and strength training. She also consulted with a dietitian to get tips on healthy eating.

After a few months of regular exercise and a healthy diet, Cynthia lost 8 kg and felt more energetic. Her physical condition and well-being improved significantly, and she gained motivation to continue taking care of her health.

Jennifer, 53 years old

Jennifer experienced severe hot flashes and difficulty sleeping. She decided to consult her doctor, who recommended hormone replacement therapy (HRT). In addition to HRT, Jennifer decided to make lifestyle changes.

She started exercising regularly, choosing mainly walking, yoga, and light strength training. She also changed her diet by incorporating more vegetables, fruits, and whole grain products. She tried to drink more water and avoid processed foods.

After a few months, Jennifer noticed a significant improvement in her well-being. She managed to lose 6 kg, and her menopausal symptoms, such as hot flashes and sleep difficulties, significantly decreased. Jennifer continues her healthy lifestyle and enjoys better health.

Tips from Experts

Dietary Tips

5. Eat a balanced diet rich in protein, healthy fats, and complex carbohydrates.
6. Avoid processed foods and simple sugars.
7. Include fiber-rich foods such as vegetables, fruits, and whole grain products in your diet.
8. Drink plenty of water to stay hydrated and support digestion.
9. Use moderate amounts of healthy fats, such as olive oil, avocado, and nuts.
10. Eat regular meals to maintain steady energy levels and avoid hunger pangs.

12. Incorporate phytoestrogens into your diet, such as soy and flaxseed, which can help alleviate menopausal symptoms.
13. Limit alcohol intake, which is high in calories and can contribute to weight gain.
14. Choose healthy snacks such as nuts, natural yogurt, and fruits to stay satisfied.
15. Ensure adequate intake of vitamins and minerals by eating a varied diet.

Fitness Tips

1. Exercise regularly to maintain a healthy weight and improve fitness.
2. Combine strength training, aerobic exercise, and stretching for the best results.
3. Start with short sessions and gradually increase the intensity and duration of your workouts.
4. Choose activities you enjoy to make it easier to stay motivated.
5. Practice relaxation techniques such as yoga and meditation to reduce stress.
6. Exercise outdoors to improve your mood and increase motivation.

7. Regularly monitor your progress to track changes and stay motivated.

8. Ensure proper warm-up before exercises and cool-down afterward.

9. Include strength training in your workout plan to increase muscle mass and boost metabolism.

10. Exercise with friends or join a fitness group to increase motivation and enjoy the activity.

Health Tips

1. Visit your doctor regularly and have check-ups to monitor your health.

2. Consult your doctor if menopausal symptoms worsen or new health problems arise.

3. Consider hormone replacement therapy (HRT) if menopausal symptoms are very troublesome.

4. Use dietary supplements such as calcium, vitamin D, and magnesium to support bone and heart health.

5. Maintain a healthy diet and regular physical activity to prevent chronic diseases.

6. Avoid stress and use relaxation techniques to improve your well-being.

7. Ensure adequate sleep to maintain health and energy.

8. Eat healthy meals and avoid processed foods to maintain

a healthy weight.

9. Use natural methods to alleviate menopausal symptoms, such as phytoestrogens and herbs.

10. Maintain a healthy body weight to prevent heart disease, type 2 diabetes, and osteoporosis.

These expert tips cover various aspects of health, from diet and fitness to mental health and overall well-being. Regularly applying these recommendations can help women during menopause effectively manage weight and improve their quality of life.

Chapter 9: FAQ

Frequently Asked Questions

1. Can you lose weight during menopause?

Yes, it is possible with the right diet and physical activity. It is crucial to understand how hormonal changes affect your body and adapt to them.

2. What supplements can help manage weight during menopause?

Consider supplements like calcium, vitamin D, magnesium, and omega-3. They can support bone and heart health and improve sleep quality.

3. Does HRT affect weight?

Hormone replacement therapy (HRT) can affect weight, but its primary goal is to alleviate menopausal symptoms. Consult your doctor to evaluate if HRT is appropriate and how it might impact your weight.

4. What are the best exercises for weight loss during menopause?

The best exercises combine strength training, aerobic exercise, and stretching. Regular walking, running, swimming, yoga, and Pilates can be very effective.

5. Is the ketogenic diet suitable for women during menopause?

The ketogenic diet can be effective for some women, but it is important to consult a doctor or dietitian before starting to ensure it is safe and appropriate for your health condition.

6. Is reducing calorie intake effective for weight loss during menopause?

Yes, reducing calorie intake can help with weight loss, but it is important to do so in a healthy and balanced way to avoid nutritional deficiencies.

7. How to deal with hunger pangs during menopause?

Regular meals, consuming protein and fiber, drinking plenty of water, and avoiding processed foods can help control hunger pangs.

8. Does drinking alcohol affect weight during menopause?

Yes, alcohol is high in calories and can contribute to weight gain. Limiting alcohol consumption can help manage weight.

9. How important is sleep for weight loss during menopause?

Sleep quality is very important. Insufficient sleep can lead to hormonal imbalances and increased appetite, making weight loss more difficult.

10. Does stress affect weight gain during menopause?

Yes, stress can increase cortisol levels, a stress hormone that promotes fat accumulation, especially around the abdomen.

11. What are the best sources of protein for women during menopause?

Lean meats, fish, eggs, dairy, legumes, and nuts are excellent sources of protein.

12. Does drinking coffee affect weight during menopause?

Coffee can boost metabolism, but excessive caffeine intake can also increase cortisol levels. It is important to drink coffee in moderation.

13. Are cardio exercises effective for women during menopause?

Yes, cardio exercises like running, cycling, and swimming are effective in burning calories and improving cardiovascular fitness.

14. Can you increase muscle mass during menopause?

Yes, regular strength training can help increase muscle mass, which boosts metabolism and helps manage weight.

15. What foods should be avoided during menopause?

Processed foods, simple sugars, trans fats, and alcohol are foods to limit or avoid.

16. Does drinking water affect weight loss during menopause?

Yes, drinking plenty of water can help maintain hydration, improve metabolism, and reduce hunger.

17. How important is fiber in the diet of women during menopause?

Fiber aids digestion, helps maintain satiety, and regulates blood sugar levels, which is beneficial for weight management.

18. Does menopause affect insulin and blood sugar levels?

Yes, hormonal changes during menopause can affect insulin and blood sugar levels, increasing the risk of insulin resistance.

19. Is intermittent fasting suitable during menopause?

Intermittent fasting can be effective for some women, but it is important to consult a doctor before starting such a dietary regimen.

20. What are the best forms of relaxation for women during menopause?

Meditation, yoga, deep breathing, massages, and hobbies are effective forms of relaxation.

21. Is calcium and vitamin D supplementation necessary during menopause?

Calcium and vitamin D supplementation can be beneficial for bone health, but it is important to consult a doctor before starting supplementation.

22. Is a vegetarian or vegan diet suitable for women during menopause?

Yes, a well-balanced vegetarian or vegan diet that provides all necessary nutrients can be suitable.

23. Are outdoor exercises better than indoor exercises?

Outdoor exercises can improve mood and increase motivation, but both types of exercise are beneficial.

24. Docs menopause affect the cardiovascular system?

Yes, a drop in estrogen levels can increase the risk of heart disease. Regular exercise and a healthy diet can help protect the heart.

25.   How to deal with fatigue during menopause?

Regular exercise, a healthy diet, adequate sleep, and relaxation techniques can help combat fatigue.

26.   Does menopause affect mental health?

Hormonal changes can affect mood and mental health. Emotional support, relaxation techniques, and therapy can be helpful.

27.   What are effective methods for managing hot flashes?

Wearing light clothing, avoiding hot drinks and spicy foods, regular exercise, and relaxation techniques can help manage hot flashes.

28.   Are there natural methods to alleviate menopausal symptoms?

Yes, phytoestrogens, herbs like black cohosh, and techniques like acupuncture can help alleviate menopausal symptoms.

29.   How important is social support during menopause?

Social support can help cope with stress and emotions, improving overall well-being.

30.   Does menopause affect thyroid function?

Hormonal changes can affect the thyroid. It is important to monitor thyroid function and consult a doctor if symptoms like fatigue, weight gain, or mood swings occur.

Thank You for Your Purchase!

c

Dear Valued Customer,

Thank you for purchasing "Menopause Weight Loss for Women"! As a small publisher, your feedback is incredibly valuable. Please consider leaving a review to help us improve our products. Your support is crucial for our growth. Thank you for choosing us!

Warm regards,

Daphne Sinclair

For your convenience, the QR code takes you directly to the review page :)

www.ingramcontent.com/pod-product-compliance
Lightning Source LLC
Chambersburg PA
CBHW061056250726
48653CB00001B/425